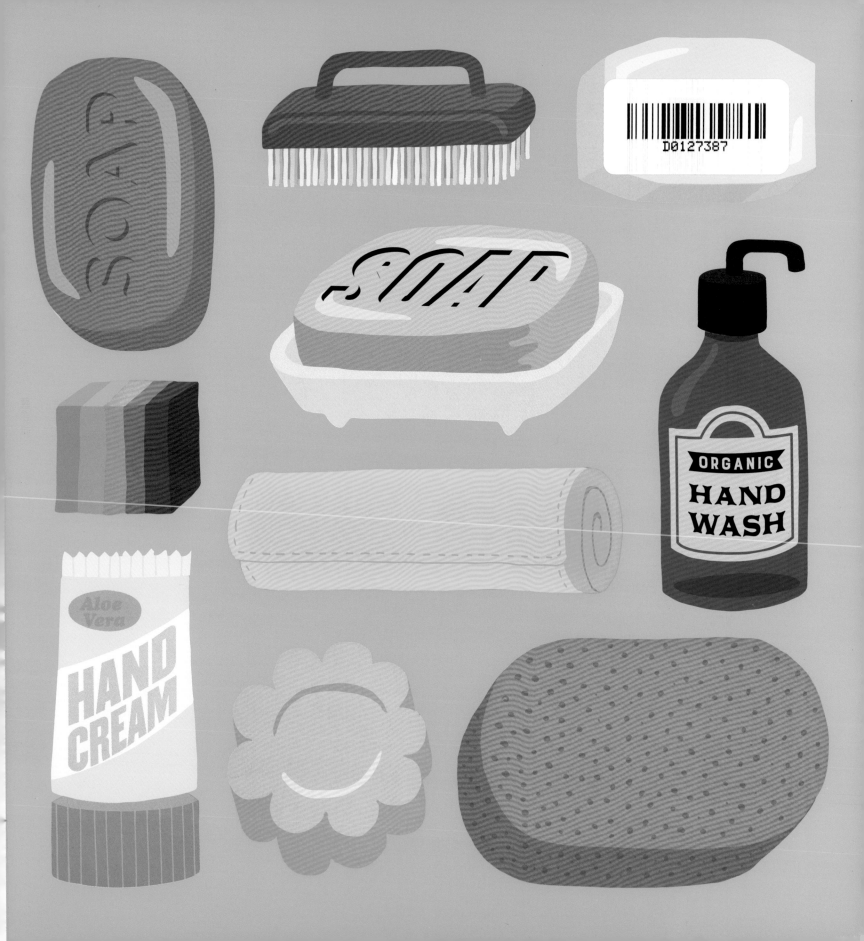

For Coco, Mabel, Delilah and Ivy — M.C.
Dedicated to the amazing people who work for the NHS!

First published in the United Kingdom in
2020 by Scholastic Children's Books

Library of Congress Cataloging-in-Publication Data Available

ISBN 978-1-338-73426-3

10 9 8 7 6 5 4 3 2 1   20 21 22 23 24

Printed in China   153
This edition first printing, October 2020

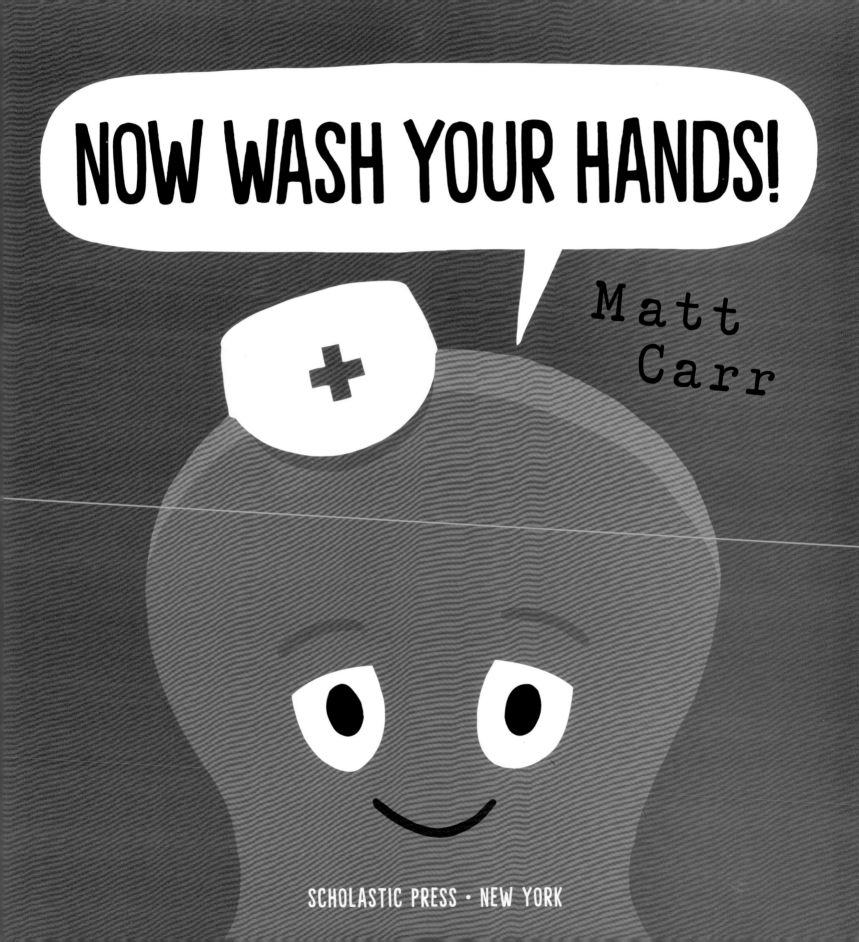

At school the kids
were running wild,
the thing that
kids do best . . .

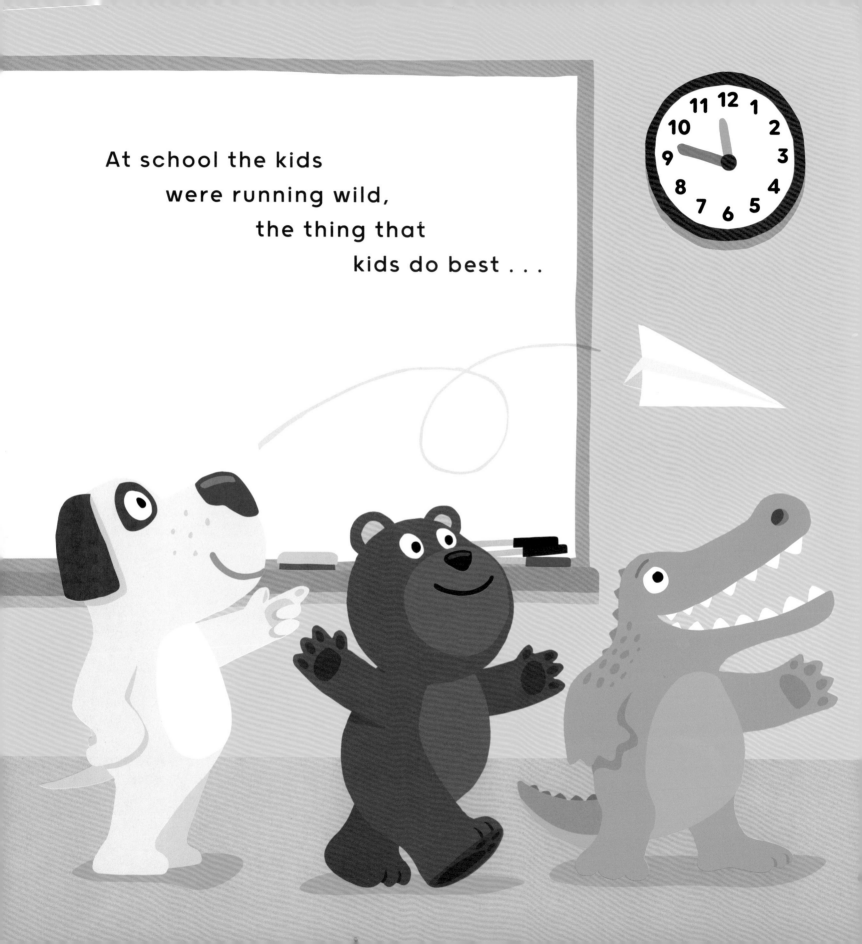

When Mrs. Moo came in the room with a very special guest.

"Doctorpus Doris
is here today,
for a really
important chat.
So make sure that
you're listening
and sitting on
the mat!"

I ♥ TEA-CHING!

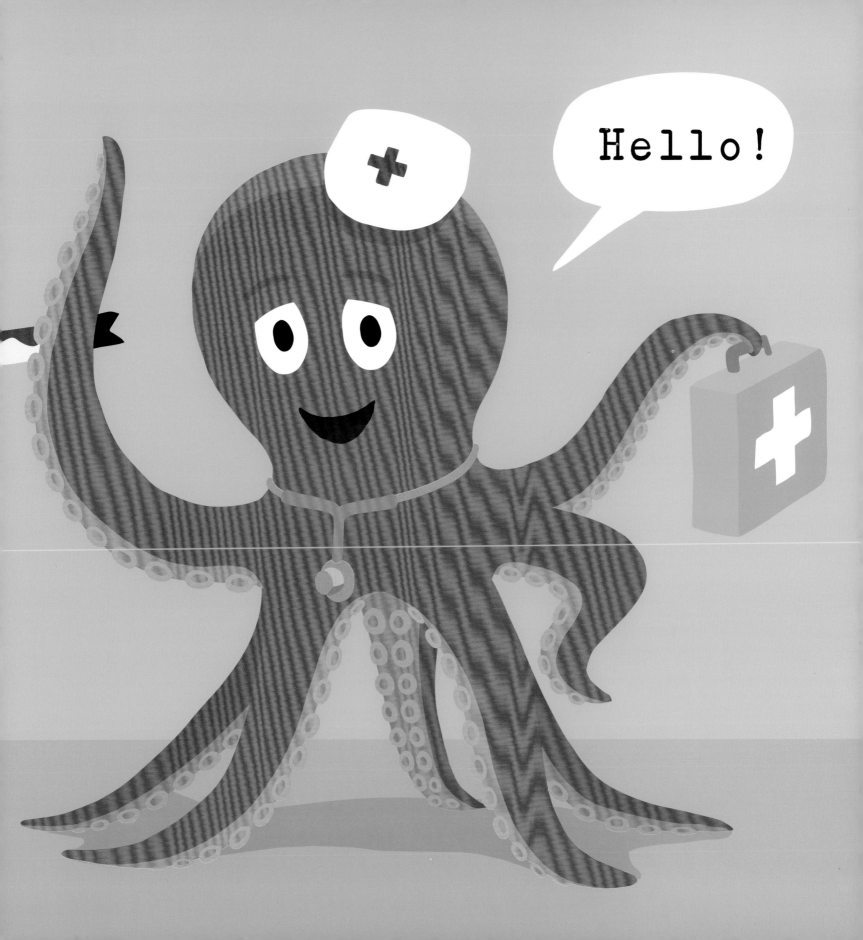

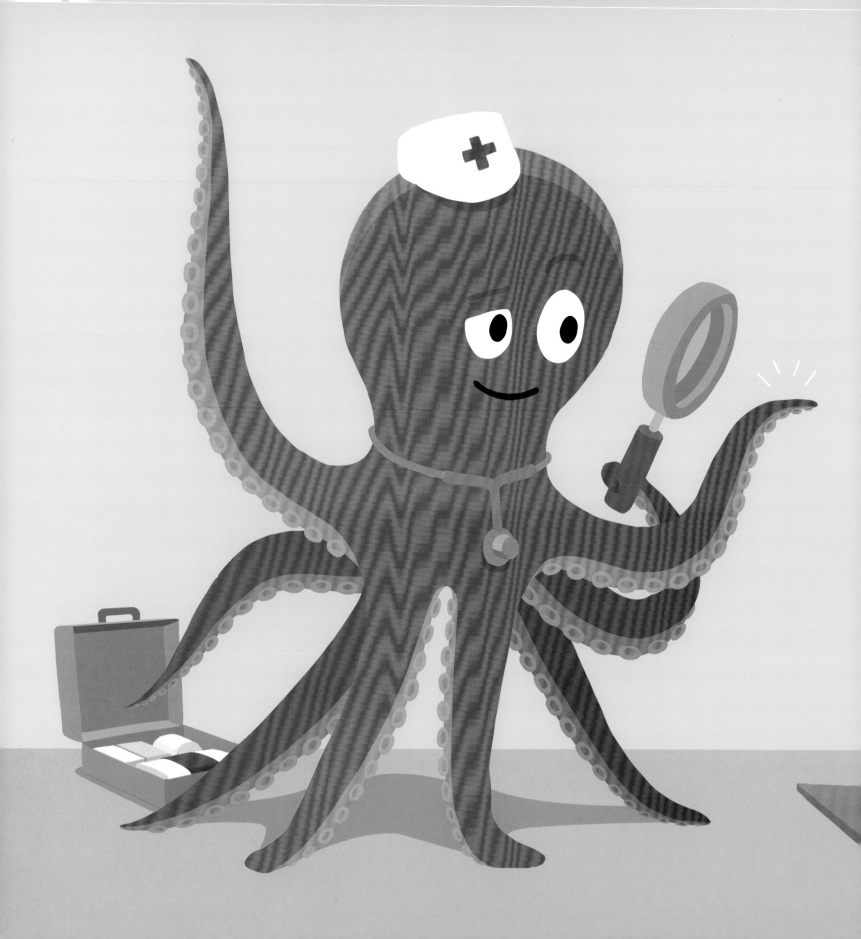

"I'd like to tell you all about
something VERY, VERY small.

In fact they are so TEENY WEENY,
you can't see them at all!"

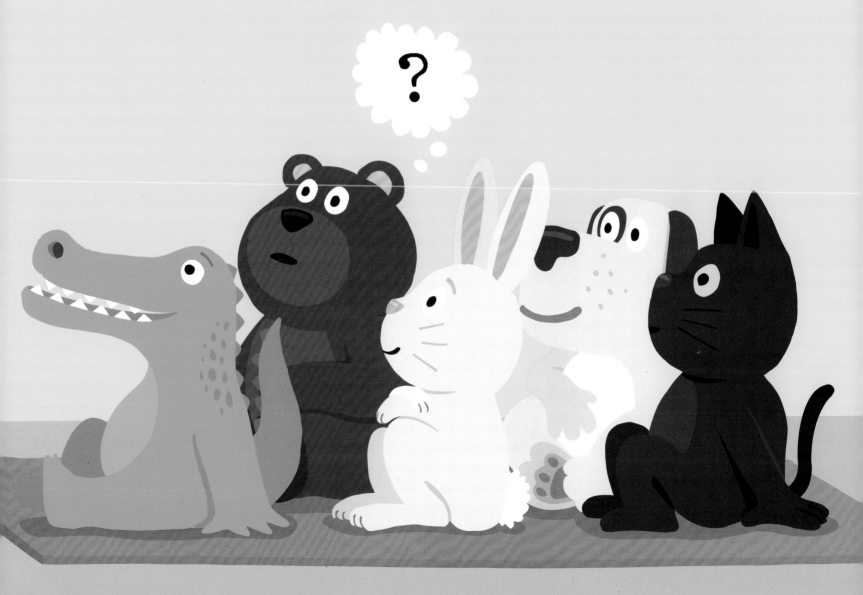

"We like to call them **GERMS!** And it's you they want to hug . . .

We love you!

. . . But the only trouble is, they can give you a nasty bug!"

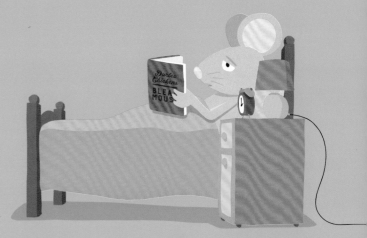

"How many **GERMS** would fit on this spoon?"

The first paw in the air was William's . . .

"Is it about one hundred?" he asked . . .

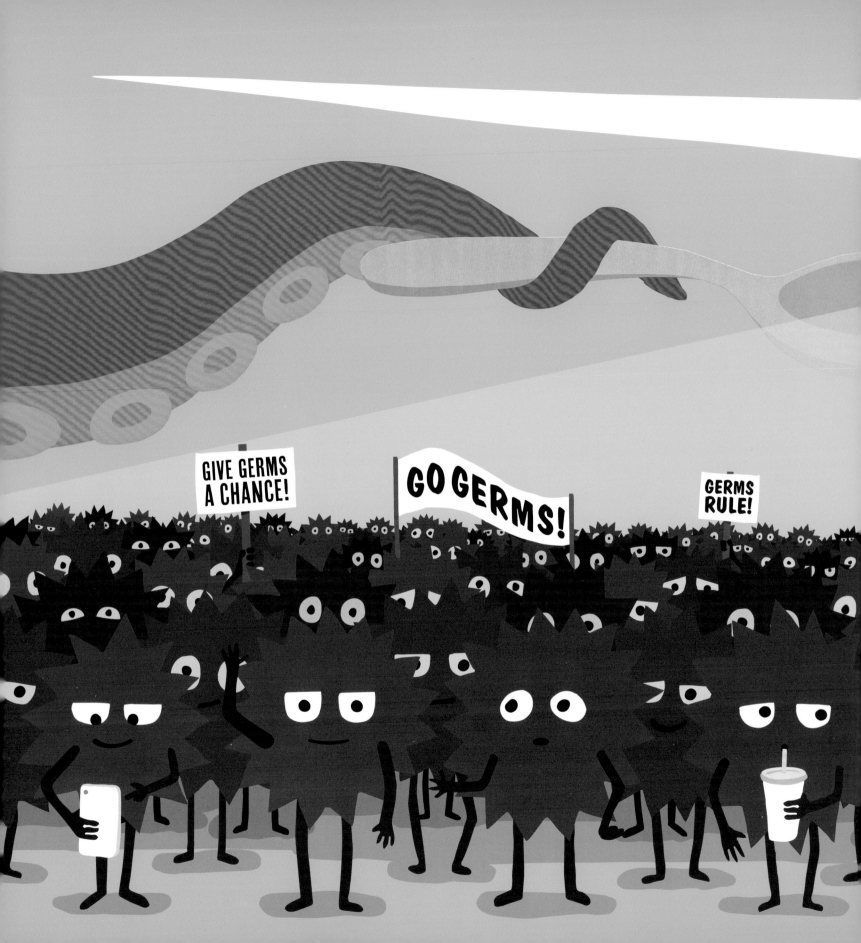

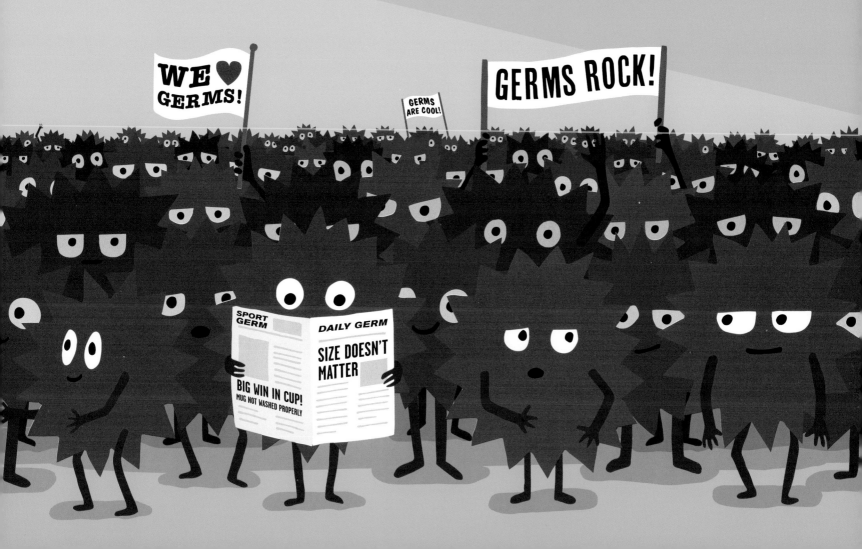

"But the good news is, there's a simple thing
that little germs can't stand . . .

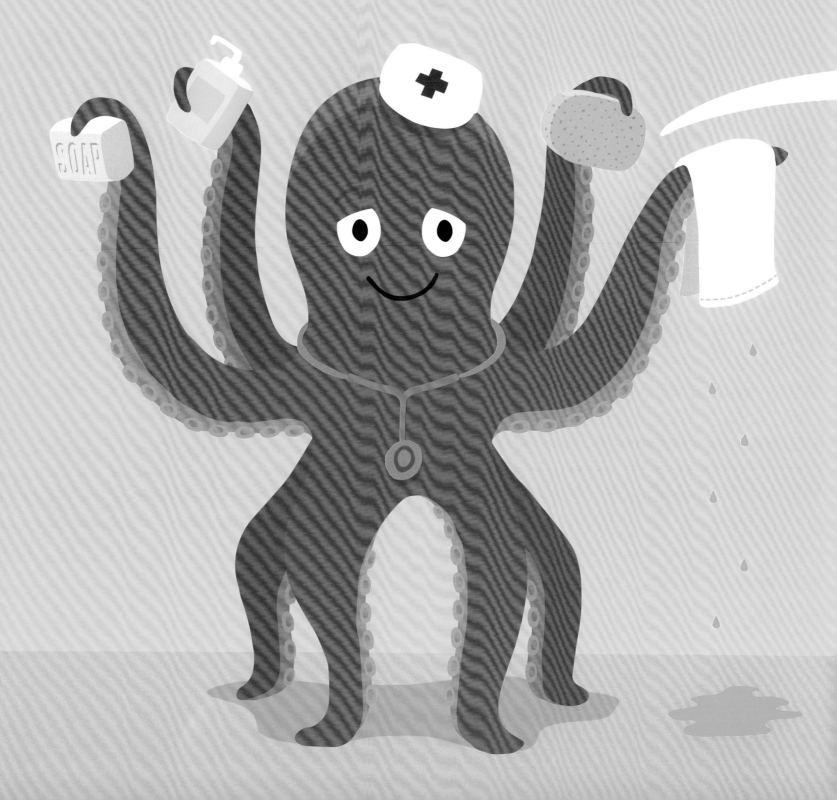

If you don't want them
to hang around, all you do is . . .

WASH YOUR HANDS!"

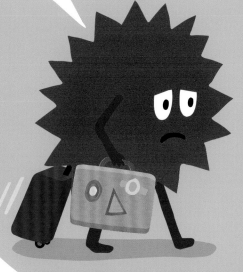

"When you've been down on the farm, Mabel, playing with the lambs. Do you know what you need to do next?"

"Yes, you WASH YOUR HANDS!"

"Or if you're in the garden with Mom, potting up some plants . . ."

COMPOST

"You **WASH YOUR HANDS** when you get inside."

"Don't give those germs a chance!"

"And, Kenny, what about in the bathroom, when you've gone PEE or POO?"

"Do you **WASH YOUR HANDS,** Doctor?"

DOG QUIXOT
MIGUEL DE CERVANTES

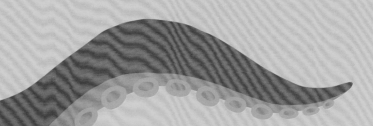

"**YES!** It's the only thing to do!"

The lunch bell rang in the classroom; the kids began to stand . . .

"But what do we do before we eat our food?"

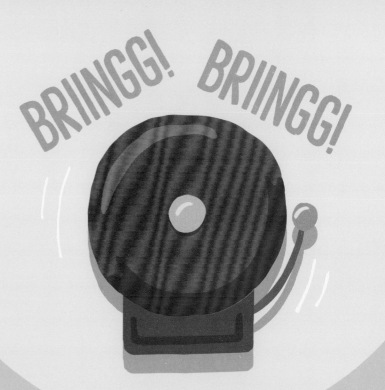

BRIINGG! BRIINGG!

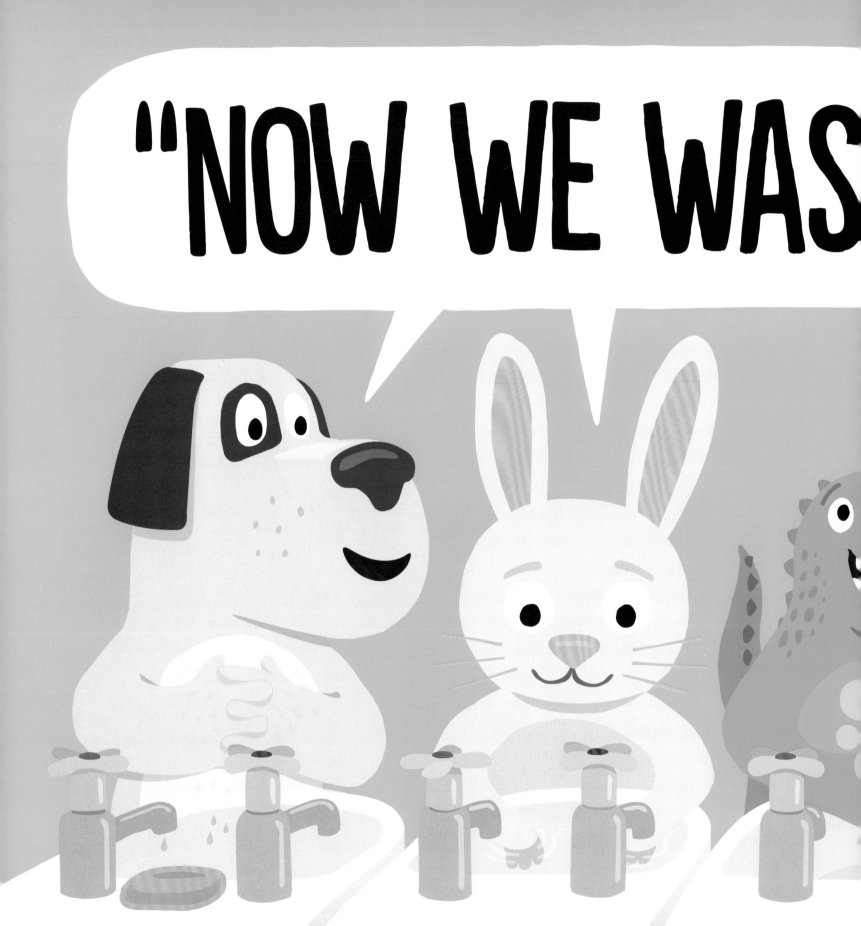

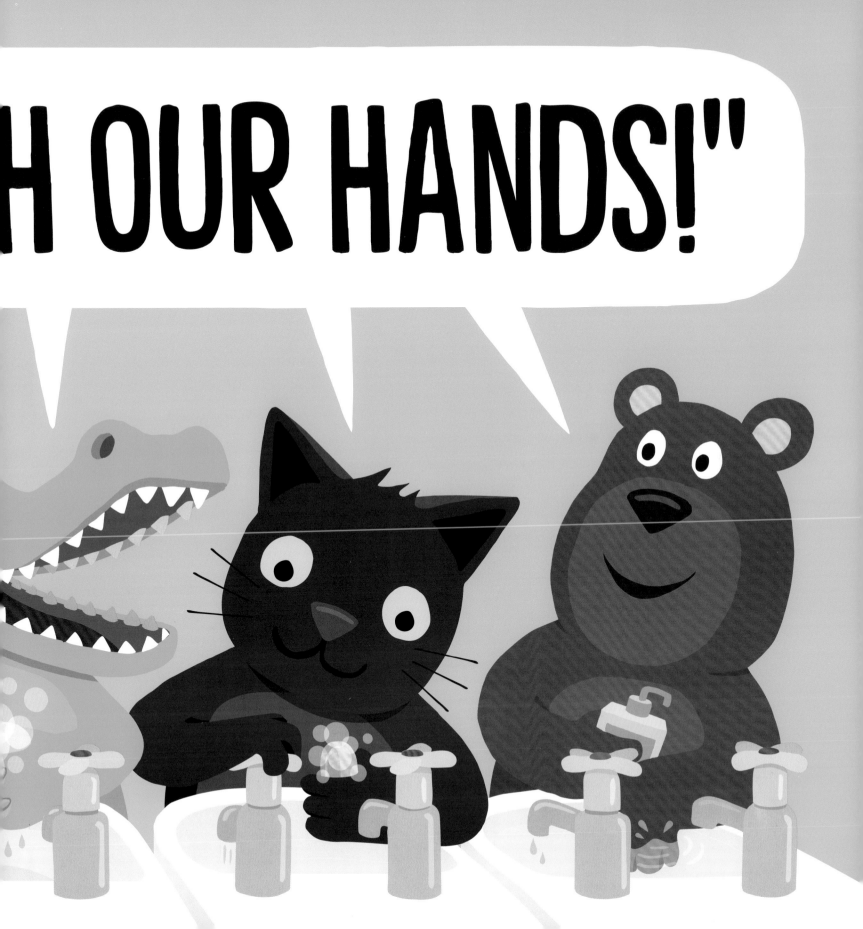

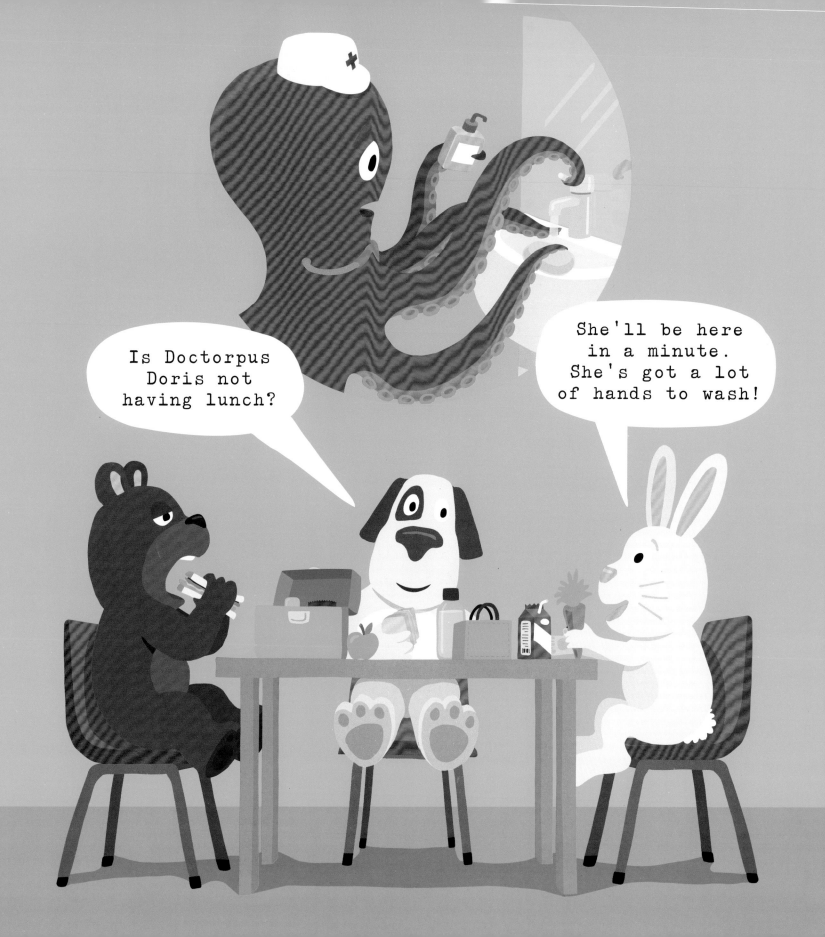

DORIS'S HANDY HAND-WASHING SONG!

WASH YOUR HANDS, it's EASY,

WASH YOUR HANDS, it's FUN.

WASH YOUR HANDS

so you don't

pass on GERMS to anyone!

Use lots of SOAP and WATER,

Then DRY them when

you're done.

It's the SIMPLE way

to KEEP GERMS AT BAY,

WASH YOUR HANDS, EVERYONE!

Sing this when you wash your hands to help you give them a super scrub!

GIVE YOUR PAWS A PROPER PAMPER!

Palm to palm

Back of your hands

Between your fingers

Back of your fingers

Fingertips

Don't forget your thumbs!

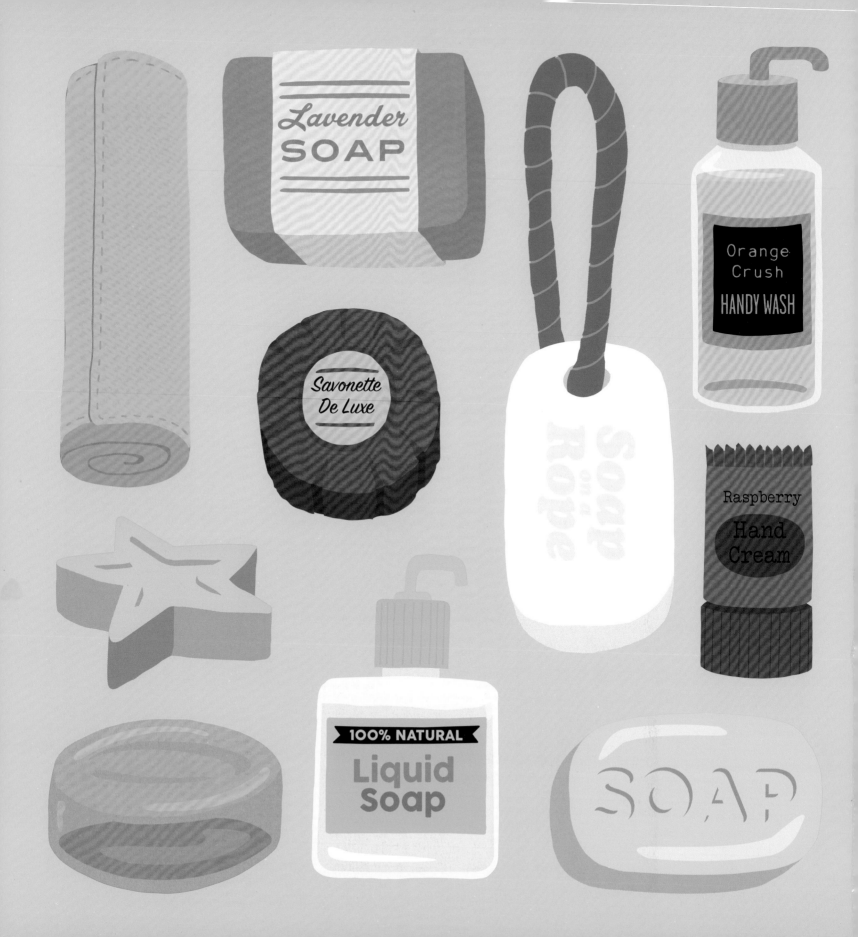